HEROES OF CANCER
PREVENTION
RESEARCH

How scientists are discovering the environmental factors

that increase the risk of cancer and how to overcome them.

July 2012

RICHARD L. HANSLER, PH.D.

ISBN: 1477662081
ISBN-13: 9781477662083

Library of Congress Control Number: 2012910924
CreateSpace
North Charleston, SC

DEDICATION

To women everywhere who can reduce their risk of breast cancer
by learning from the discoveries
by the scientists described in this
book. And to men who can reduce
their risk of prostate cancer in the
same way.

PREFACE

This book honors scientists who have contributed significantly to understanding the daily rhythms in living things, how these rhythms are controlled, and how they affect health. It is based on my study of their peer reviewed technical papers published in respected journals. This task was made possible in large part due to the database maintained by the US government that abstracts medical journals and contains more than 40 million abstracts. It is available to everyone on the web at http://www.pubmed.gov. Many of the abstracts provide links to free copies of the entire paper. I suggest that if you see some item of particular interest, you look it up on PubMed.

INDEX

INTRODUCTION

The cure rate for cancer is gradually improving, but is still far from impressive, especially if the cancer is not discovered in its early stages. Early detection is helpful, but recent studies indicate that for younger women, screening for breast cancer using mammography is not having any significant effect on mortality. For this reason it is becoming a more widely held view that "Prevention Is the Cure." To this end we see more and more articles that talk about eating healthy diets, with emphasis on the benefits of antioxidants. However, again the statistics are not very impressive. There is no question that eating less red meat, switching to low-fat foods, and limiting alcohol intake is helpful in reducing cancer. We know the cancer rate is much lower in primitive societies that don't have all our "advanced" technology. In this book we are honoring research scientists who are looking at what else in our environment can we modify to reduce the risk of cancer, especially breast and prostate cancer. Their findings suggest some changes in lifestyle you may want to try in order to reduce your risks.

CHAPTER 1
Eva Schernhammer, MD, PhD

I read somewhere that one of the heroes of cancer prevention research, Dr. Eva Schernhammer, developed her interest in breast cancer research when a number of her friends, who were nurses, developed the dread disease. She wondered if it had anything to do with their having to work at night. When she arrived at Harvard, with ready access to the Nurses' Health Study, she figured out how to get an answer. What she found provided the motivation for my work. On the web page of Harvard's Channing Laboratory, where she works, she describes her research interests (in part) as follows:

> My primary research interest is in exploring the exposures that influence the circadian system in humans. I have done work on the effects of light at night on cancer risk through the melatonin pathway and demonstrated that the effects of light at night may affect not only breast cancer, but also other cancers such as colorectal cancer, generating evidence that supports a new hypothesis on the development of cancer. I have also conducted urinary melatonin measurements in the Nurses' Health Study (see below) to assess the hormone's variations according to shift work status and its association with breast cancer risk in the Nurses' Health Study.

On a different page of the Website for Harvard's Channing Laboratory it describes the Nurses' Health Studies as follows:

> The Nurses' Health Studies are among the largest and longest-running investigations of factors that influence

women's health. Started in 1976 and expanded in 1989, the information provided by the 238,000 dedicated nurse-participants has led to many new insights on health and disease. While the prevention of cancer is still a primary focus, the study has also produced landmark data on cardiovascular disease, diabetes, and many other conditions. Most importantly, these studies have shown that diet, physical activity, and other lifestyle factors can powerfully promote better health.

In 2001 Dr. Schernhammer published a milestone paper in which she established that nurses who had worked rotating shifts for many years had a significantly higher risk of breast cancer than those who had not worked rotating shifts. She did this by sorting through the records of the tens of thousands of nurses who had participated in this study to find those who had worked rotating shifts for many years. She then found a similar group of the same age, habits, etc. that had not worked rotating shifts for many years. Next she looked at how many in each group had been diagnosed with breast cancer. From this data she calculated how much more likely one group was to have breast cancer than the other group. The odds ratio for those who had worked more than 15 years on rotating shifts was 1.35. Said another way, their chance of getting breast cancer was 35% greater than for those who had never worked rotating shifts. Said still another way, if you had equal-size groups of nurses who had worked rotating shifts for more than 15 years and those that had not, if 100 in the "had not" group developed breast cancer, then in the group that "had" worked rotating shifts, there would be 135 who developed breast cancer. Since this result was for a very large number of nurses, it was especially meaningful. The chance of this increased cancer incidence being just by chance was less than one in one thousand. Because many people work rotating shifts, this paper generated a lot of attention. It appeared in 2001 with the title, "Rotating Night Shifts and Risk of Breast Cancer in Women Participating in the Nurses' Health Study." It had a total of five authors besides Schernhammer. This was a stunning way to launch her career at Harvard. In the ten years following this study, she appeared as an author on 58 papers in technical journals. Of these, 34 concerned cancer and 24 breast cancer. We will stay focused on breast cancer.

There must have been a lot of speculation concerning the cause of this elevated rate of breast cancer resulting from rotating-shift work. Many other scientists had been observing the effect of light on animals. They found that exposing them to light at night, which resulted in suppression of melatonin, caused a higher incidence of breast cancers. They also found that exposing them to light at night accelerated the growth rate of tumors. Dr. Richard Stevens, whom we will be discussing in chapter 5, proposed what came to be known as the "Melatonin Hypothesis." He attributes the increased incidence of cancer to the loss of melatonin, due to the use of light at night. In 2004 Schernhammer published a paper in which she proposed that it was probably the reduction in the flow of melatonin that was responsible for the elevated risk of breast cancer for nurses working rotating shifts for many years. She posed it as a question in the title of the paper "Melatonin and Cancer Risk: Does Light at Night Compromise Physiologic Cancer Protection by Lowering Serum Melatonin Levels?"

Dr. Schernhammer's next related effort was to try to see if it was stress associated with caregiving that might be causing the elevated breast cancer rate for nurses working rotating shifts. This study found no evidence that caregiving resulted in an increased risk of breast cancer.

Her next breast cancer–related study was a logical extension of the melatonin hypothesis. If low melatonin as a result of shift work was causing cancer, then women with breast cancer would probably be found to be producing less melatonin at night. By collecting overnight urine and looking for the metabolite (residue) of melatonin in overnight urine, the answer could be found. She did, in fact, find that women with invasive breast cancer did produce urine overnight with less of the melatonin metabolite. She concluded women who make less melatonin are more likely to get breast cancer. Other scientists who had done similar studies interpreted the results in a different way. Some said that as a result of the cancer, the women produced less melatonin. At least one study found that the early stage of breast cancer stimulated melatonin production but that as the cancer grew, the melatonin production dropped off.

Because the earlier study had looked at the increased risk of breast cancer for women working rotating shifts, Dr. Schernhammer went back and did another study looking at night work and breast cancer. She also looked at other similar studies in other countries. Her conclusion was that there was substantial evidence that working night shift resulted in an increased incidence of breast cancer and probably some other cancers as well.

If melatonin was so important in protecting women from cancer, were there foods that contained melatonin, or the material from which melatonin is produced, that could protect from cancer? She looked at what the nurses in the study ate and looked for some correlation with who got breast cancer. The results of this study were negative. Nothing seemed to be of much benefit. What did appear was that eating red meat increased the risk of breast and some other cancers.

One of the most brilliant studies she did was to make use of a measurement of melatonin metabolite in overnight urine done as part of the Nurses' Health Study. The sample-givers were divided into four groups in the order of their concentration of melatonin metabolite. Of the large number of nurses who had provided these samples, a certain number developed breast cancer over the course of the next eight years. Of the fourth of the nurses who had produced the highest concentration of melatonin metabolite, the chance of developing breast cancer was only 60% compared to the fourth of the nurses who had the lowest concentration of melatonin residue. This is further evidence that maximizing melatonin provides protection from breast cancer. It also partially answers the question of whether having breast cancer lowers melatonin or having lower melatonin increases risk of getting cancer. This experiment says the latter is true. It doesn't say whether the former may also be true.

One of the earliest indications that light at night might contribute to breast cancer was a 1991 study by epidemiologist R. Hahn who found that blind women had a much lower incidence of breast cancer than women with normal vision. Dr. Schernhammer extended this idea in an interesting way. It is known that some blind women who have no vision still respond to light that controls their internal clock, their circadian rhythm, and their production of melatonin. She looked at the incidence of breast cancer in these two different groups of blind women. She found, as one would expect, that the women who were totally blind had a lower rate of breast cancer than those who still responded to light.

In a 2009 paper, Dr. Schernhammer enumerates the many ways in which melatonin is able to fight against breast and other cancers. It is a powerful antioxidant that can destroy damaged DNA before it can initiate cancer, it prevents cell mobility that is the cause of the spread of cancer to distant sites (metastasis), it prevents the growth of blood vessels that provide nourishment for cancer, it modulates the immune system, it alters fat metabolism, and it blocks the ability of estrogen to promote cancer growth. The abstract of the paper states, "As evidence increases, modifiable factors that have been shown to affect melatonin production, such as night shift work, are likely to gain increasing recognition as potential public health hazards." This suggests (probably inadvertently) that those who are not night-shift workers are immune from the damage of light at night. Nothing is farther from the truth, and I doubt it was her intent to imply that. This is unfortunate, since virtually all people in advanced societies suffer the bad effects of light at night. What is curious is the reluctance on the part of researchers to say that light at night is bad.. The only thing I can think of is that they are always in need of funding to continue their studies. If they come right out and say that light at night is bad and is killing people, then there is less need for more studies. Fortunately the reader does not need their endorsement to take action.

Summary of Dr. Schernhammer's most significant conclusions:

1. Women (both pre- and post-menopausal) who have worked night shift for a long time (more than 15 years) have a higher risk of breast cancer than women who have not worked night shift..

2. Women who have breast cancer have a lower concentration of the melatonin metabolite in overnight urine than women who do not have breast cancer.

3. Women who produce the most melatonin during the night have a much lower (60%) risk of breast cancer than women who produce the least melatonin during the night.

4. There are a significant number of ways that melatonin fights breast and endometrial cancers.

5. Totally blind women have a lower incidence of breast cancer than blind women who still perceive light enough to control the circadian cycle. This means they have reduced production of melatonin due to exposure to light at night required by family members with normal vision.

Dr. Schernhammer's studies provide very convincing evidence that maximizing melatonin production will reduce the risk of breast (and other) cancer.

CHAPTER 2
David E. Blask, PhD, MD

The following statement, copied from the Tulane University web page, is a concise statement of why Dr. Blask should be considered one of the heroes of cancer prevention research.

> Dr. David Blask, a widely acclaimed expert on cancer biology, circadian rhythms, and the health implications of exposure to light at night, has joined Tulane University School of Medicine as a professor of practice in the Department of Structural and Cellular Biology.
>
> In the early 1980s, Blask was one of only a handful of scientists studying regulation of breast cancer development and growth by melatonin, a hormone produced by the pineal gland (a small pine cone–shaped gland located near the center of the brain) during sleep in the darkness of night. Melatonin modulates many of the body's natural circadian rhythms, or the daily cycle of biological activity during a 24-hour period, including the sleep/wake cycle. Melatonin has been shown to have important anti-cancer properties.
>
> "This was considered fringe science at the time and several colleagues warned that pursuing this area of study would be a career breaker," Blask says.
>
> However, his lab at the University of Arizona was the first to demonstrate that nighttime blood levels of melatonin directly suppress human breast cancer cell growth. Dr. Steven Hill, current Structural and Cellular Biology chair,

was a graduate student in Blask's lab at the time and performed these groundbreaking experiments.

"It was one of those 'Eureka' moments that don't come too often in one's career," Blask said. Since then, he has become a world-renowned expert on the negative health implications and increased cancer risk associated with melatonin suppression due to exposure to light at night.

Using specially designed photoperiodic chambers, which allow precise control over light exposure at night, he and his research team were the first to demonstrate that manipulating light intensity at night, and thus melatonin production, dramatically affects human breast cancers growing in rats. Their experiments showed that reduced levels of melatonin caused by brighter intensities of light at night boosted human breast cancer tumor growth in rats.

This landmark research helped to lay the groundwork for a scientific working group (of which Blask was a member) appointed by the World Health Organization to add shift work and exposure to light at night to its list of possible carcinogens. Shift workers have been shown to have higher risks for breast, prostate and other cancers.

Blask was also recently invited to brief a group of Congressional staffers on the implications of light pollution on the environment in June as part of an effort to get the Environmental Protection Agency to address the problem.

"Dr. Blask's arrival will help us to further develop our efforts to build a center of excellence in circadian melatonin cancer biology," said Hill, who hopes to add additional scientists to his team in the near future. "There is only one other group in the United States working in this area. As we continue to recruit the best and brightest in this field, Tulane is in a position to become the world's premiere center for research into cancer chronotherapy and prevention."

Dr. Blask's published studies of breast cancer began in 1986 when he reported the results on an experiment in which rats were injected with a drug (a carcinogen) to cause development of mammary tumors (breast cancer). Two treatments were tested: one consisted of a 30% reduction of food and the second was an injection of melatonin. Each treatment reduced the incidence and growth rate of tumors, but the combination was most effective. I haven't heard of a reduction of food as a treatment for human breast cancer. There is evidence that obesity is a risk factor for breast cancer.

He next reported on experiments in which cancer cells of the type that were stimulated to grow by estrogen were cultured in a dish and treated with melatonin. At a melatonin concentration similar to that in the body at night, the cells stopped growing. At either higher or lower concentrations of melatonin, the cells started growing again.

In his first reported study (1990) of the effect of light on melatonin production, he was working with rats. Rats' eyes are enormously more sensitive to light than human eyes. He showed they also have remarkably greater sensitivity to melatonin-suppressing light. He found that during a time when melatonin was normally flowing, just exposing the rats to dim light greatly increased the growth of tumors. The role of linoleic acid in cancer progression was also established. Interfering with the metabolism of linoleic acid is one of the mechanisms by which melatonin suppresses tumor growth.

In another study, mammary cancers were produced in rats by injecting a carcinogen. Treatment consisted of injections of melatonin and of 9-cis-retinoic acid. Of the animals that received no treatment, 55% developed tumors. Of those that received both melatonin and 9-cis-retinoic acid, 5% developed tumors. The number rose to 20% for those treated only every other day. Time for tumors to develop was also increased in the treated animals. This appears to be a potent combination.

The group that Dr. Blask was working with had learned how to graft human breast cancer tumors to the backs of rats. In this study, human breast cancer tumors of the type known to respond to estrogen were grafted to rats. Some rats were living under constant light and some under an alternating light-dark schedule. Under the light-dark schedule, they had a robust melatonin rhythm. Under constant light, they produced almost no melatonin. The tumors on the constant-light animals grew much faster than the ones in the light-dark group. The metabolism of linoleic acid by the tumors was measured and found to be much faster in the constant-light group. This (to my knowledge) is the first direct experimental evidence (rather than epidemiological) of the link between light exposure that suppresses melatonin, and human breast cancer.

A milestone paper with 13 authors was published in 2005 that was probably the main reason the World Health Organization decided to classify night-shift work that disrupted the circadian rhythm as a "probable carcinogen." In this study, human breast cancer tumors known to be stimulated by estrogen were grafted to rats but supplied with human blood. They found that human blood drawn at night, when the donors had been exposed to light and therefore lacked melatonin, caused rapid growth of human breast cancers grafted to rats. Blood from these donors that was drawn during the day, when they were exposed to light, caused rapid growth of the cancers. The blood from the same donors drawn in darkness (and which therefore contained melatonin) did not stimulate cancer growth. Dr. Blask described the effect of melatonin as putting the cancers to sleep.

The most recent study (2009) using this same technique broadened the results of an earlier study to include estrogen-receptor-negative (ER-) breast cancers (which are not stimulated by estrogen) with a similar result. The mechanism was shown to be the inhibition of the metabolism of linoleic acid into a substance (13-HODE) that causes mitosis (cell division). ER- grafts on rats exposed to light grew more rapidly than on rats on a light-dark schedule. Experiments where the grafts were fed with human blood, when the blood was from donors subjected to a brief exposure to bright light, grew rapidly as well. The stated conclusion is most relevant and says in part, "this mechanism partially explains the higher risk of breast cancer for…those who experience prolonged exposure to light at night" (everyone). Because the effect of light at night was originally found in night-shift workers, people dismiss it as not relating to them. **Everyone is subject to light at night and suffers the same negative result as night-shift workers.**

Summary of Dr. Blask's studies:

1. In his early studies of animals, he established the connection between prolonged light exposure, loss of melatonin, and stimulated growth of cancer.

2. By studying cultured estrogen positive cancer cells, he established the relationship between the stimulating effects of estrogen and the way melatonin blocks that effect.

3. He found that an agent (HODE) that causes cell division (mitosis) is produced when cancer cells use linoleic acid as a food. This leads to metastasis of the cancer. Melatonin blocks this process.

4. He, along with Brainard and others, demonstrated that human cancers grown on the backs of rats but supplied with human blood grew rapidly when the blood lacked melatonin and slowly when it contained melatonin.

5. He showed that only a relatively brief exposure to light during the night results in a marked reduction in the amount of melatonin produced.

6. These experiments were important factors which resulted in the World Health Organization classifying light at night, which causes circadian disruption, as a probable carcinogen.

Two names that appear most frequently with that of Dr. Blask are Robert Dauchy and Leonard Sauer. These two were studying cancer in rats for a long time before Dr. Blask joined their efforts. They appeared to have developed the technique for growing human breast cancer on the backs of rats in which they could provide the tumors with human blood. They certainly need recognition for their many years of work in establishing the light-at-night breast cancer connection.

CHAPTER 3
George C. Brainard, PhD

Dr. Stevens, a professor at the University of Connecticut (see chapter 5), published a tongue-in-cheek paper titled "Electric Light Causes Cancer, Surely You're Joking, Mr. Stevens?" in which he spells out the basic argument of this book. He describes (in part) the huge contribution of Dr. Brainard in the following way:

> Bud Brainard at Jefferson Medical College had been working furiously for years to define the precise wavelengths of light that maximally suppress melatonin, as a marker of circadian rhythmicity, in the middle of the night. This spectral response function was critical to figuring out the phototransduction mechanism for the circadian system. By the late 1990s accumulating evidence was suggesting that the primary mechanism was not vision *per se*, although the retina appeared to be required. Some of this evidence was from blind persons and from retinally degenerate mice. In 2001, Bud published his spectral response and later an important extension of it to phase resetting in a study led by Steve Lockley, a very talented chronobiologist in Cziesler's lab. The melatonin response spectrum required hundreds of arduous individual experiments in which volunteers were in the lab overnight and exposed to one of many combinations of monochromatic light of a specific wavelength and a specific photon flux density. It took over 5 years to do it right. The peak sensitivity turns out to be at about 480 nm, which is the wavelength of that beautiful blue we see in the sky on a clear day at mid-morning. It is probably no coincidence from an evolutionary perspective

that the system for telling our inner self whether it is day or not is finely tuned to that wavelength. The new photoreceptive cell found in the retina, called the intrinsically photoreceptive retinal ganglion cell (ipRGC), also responds maximally to this wavelength.

Dr. Brainard has published 76 technical papers to date that are abstracted on Pubmed.gov. Of these, 48 are concerned with melatonin. However, of these, only 9 include the word cancer. He serves on the Effect of Light on Health Committee of the Illuminating Engineering Society of North America and is a consultant to NASA on lighting for space voyages.

His relevant studies began in the 1970s. He wrote a paper summarizing the research on the pineal gland which took place between 1954 and 1965. The abstract of that paper reads as follows:

> In a little more than a decade (1954–1965), the pineal gland was demonstrated to be an active neuroendocrine transducer in contrast to a functionless vestige as earlier supposed. The two major contributions which laid the groundwork for the development of modern pineal science were Kitay and Altschule's book *The Pineal Gland* (1954) and Lerner's isolation and structural work on melatonin (1958). After Lerner's discovery, biochemists, anatomists, and physiologists determined much about the structure and function of the pineal gland. In 1965, Wurtman and Axelrod tied this earlier work together by characterizing the pineal as a neuroendocrine transducer.

Dr. Brainard summarized the ten years from 1954 to 1965 as if this represented a completed story. It was his work and that of others in this book that made the 40 years from 1965 to 2005 the years when the true importance of the pineal gland would be revealed.

His early work (1980s) concerned the effect of the color, intensity, and timing of light on the production of melatonin by the pineal gland and the effect this had on reproduction, immunity, other hormones, and general health. His early work was confined to the study of animals.

In the '90s he became interested in the way in which light exposure in the morning could be used to treat seasonal affective disorder (SAD), sometimes called the winter blues. He studied how the color of the light affected the patients. Since depression is a highly subjective condition, it was difficult to quantify the results. He concluded at one point (probably wrongly) that white light was more effective in treating SAD than green light. Modern treatment is primarily done with blue LED lights that, according to his later findings, match the response of the new sensors he discovered.

It was these studies that eventually led to his major discovery that it is primarily blue light that suppresses melatonin. These studies took over five years to complete. Volunteers would stare into a uniformly lighted sphere in which the light was one precise color (wavelength) and a specified intensity. At the end of a set period of time, a sample of blood or saliva was taken for analysis for melatonin concentration. A few nights later, the process was repeated using a different color and intensity. It was in connection with these studies that he noted the large differences between individuals in the amount of melatonin produced under the same circumstances.

In 2001 he published his most significant paper, titled "Action Spectrum for Melatonin Regulation in Humans: Evidence for a Novel Circadian Photoreceptor." One of the things truly inspiring about this, that young people should keep in mind, is that a major component in the physiology of the human eye was not discovered until the twenty-first century. We tend to think that everything important is already known. This couldn't be farther from the truth. This discovery of the new sensors in the eye is what makes it possible to conveniently extend the period of melatonin flow by blocking blue light, without giving up our normal evening activities. One of the fascinating sidelights of Dr. Brainard's work was that an almost identical study was going on in the United Kingdom by Dr. Skene at the University of Surrey. The two groups got wind of the work of the other and ended up publishing on the same day. Her paper is titled "An Action Spectrum for Melatonin Suppression: Evidence for a Novel Non-rod, Non-cone Photoreceptor System in Humans." These two studies are what make it possible to say with confidence that there is a solution to the problem of using light at night. By preventing blue light from reaching the eye during the time when melatonin is flowing, its flow may be preserved.

Drs. Brainard and Skene recognized the importance of this work and both filed patent applications. The Brainard patent issued in March 2010. The Skene patent was granted in the United States and subsequently purchased by Philips. It is hard to guess their intent.

Dr. Brainard went on to discover these newly noted sensors were not uniformly distributed in the eye but mostly on the lower part of the retina. This means it is mostly the light in the upper part of the field of view that controls the circadian system. This is of course how the blue of the sky would be controlling the body. He also did a study in which he demonstrated how the exposure to blue light can reset the circadian clock, This concept had not been considered earlier. The idea of moving the circadian cycle by timely exposure to light or darkness was all new.

In 2002 he published his first paper concerning light and cancer. In the abstract of that paper, he mentions the need for the lighting industry to take note. In part it states,

> Under highly controlled exposure circumstances, less than 1 lux of monochromatic light elicited a significant suppression of nocturnal melatonin. In view of the possible link between light exposure, melatonin suppression and cancer risk, it is important to continue to identify the basic related ocular physiology. Visual performance, rather than circadian function, has been the primary focus of architectural lighting systems. It is now necessary to reevaluate lighting strategies, with consideration of circadian influences, in an effort to

maximize physiological homeostasis and health.

That same year, Brainard and Blask began joint publishing of a series of papers, which we discussed in the previous chapter, that demonstrated the direct effect of blood, with and without melatonin, on the growth of human breast cancers. In this case, blood without melatonin was obtained both during the day when it was expected to be without melatonin and during the night when the subjects had been exposed to light and therefore lacked melatonin. The studies initially were with cancers that were stimulated by estrogen but later included breast cancers that were not. These are the studies that led to classifying light at night as a probable carcinogen.

The original study of the effect of blue light in suppressing melatonin had not clearly demonstrated that the effect dropped off at the very shortest wavelength part of the visual spectrum. In a study aimed at answering that question, the measurement of the effect of 420nm and 460nm light was compared. While the 420nm light produced a suppressing effect, the effect of 460nm light was significantly stronger. In another study, he demonstrated that although red light has only a weak effect in suppressing melatonin, if sufficiently strong it will cause some suppression.

Dr. Brainard's work with astronauts was described as follows on a website for biology teachers:

> George Brainard, a neuroscientist working with the
> National Space Biological Research Institute (NSBRI),
> is researching circadian rhythms and space flight.
> Brainard describes his work with lighting systems, which
> may help to improve the quality of astronauts' sleep
> and improve their daily performance in space. Light,
> enriched in the blue end of the spectrum, appears to
> help maintain circadian rhythms and regular sleep cycles
> in space. This research could aid people on Earth who
> experience circadian rhythm irregularities, such as those
> caused by seasonal affective disorder. Circadian rhythms

are approximate 24-hour behavioral, physiological or molecular cycles in living organisms regulated by an internal biological clock.

In an ABC Television program in which Dr. Brainard and Dr. Schernhammer were interviewed, they talked about the alarming increase in breast cancer and the effect of light at night. While reluctant to alarm people, Dr. Brainard did make the following statement:

"So if you're relaxing and you're going to bed in the evening and you're a day worker, you would not want a bright bedside lamp while you're reading a book before you go to bed, you would want something that was a softer light—a warmer light—something that is more shifted to the yellow end of the spectrum."

Summary:

1. Dr. Brainard's most significant contribution to science is his discovery of a new sensor in the retina of the eye that controls the circadian rhythm and with it the flow of melatonin. This discovery, that it is primarily the blue rays that cause melatonin suppression, is the basis of my work in developing lighting-related products that don't suppress melatonin.

2. His extensive study of the effect of light on melatonin production and tumor growth provided the incentive for him to figure out the mechanism behind it.

3. His studies of the effect of melatonin-containing blood on human cancers grown on animals (that he did in collaboration with Dr. Blask and others) led to the classification by the World Health Organization of shift work which involves circadian disruption as a probable carcinogen.

CHAPTER 4
Hella and Christian Bartsch (both PhDs)

The Bartsch family is a husband-and-wife team of scientists who have been studying the pineal gland for many years dating back to the 1980s. They are on the faculty at Tubingen University in Germany. In 2001 they organized a meeting of the leading scientists studying the circadian cycle and the pineal gland and how it impacts human breast cancer and other cancers. They published the proceedings of that conference in the book *Pineal Gland and Cancer* (Springer). While quite technical, any person serious about avoiding cancer would find this book of great interest. The Bartsches have been strong supporters of the idea of blocking blue light with amber glasses to advance the circadian cycle to an earlier time and thereby maximize the amount of melatonin produced.

Their earliest paper (1981) concerned the effect on tumors of when light was present in the circadian cycle, and how injection of melatonin had different effects on tumors, depending on when during the circadian cycle it was injected. One might say correctly that they were among the first to study chronotherapy (treatments done at a particular time in the circadian cycle).

In the '90s they did a series of experiments looking for a linkage between both breast and prostate cancer and melatonin. They raised the question, "Does having cancer reduce the amount of melatonin produced, or does having low melatonin increase the likelihood of developing cancer?" They found evidence of the former but did not rule out the latter. They established that the low melatonin in cancer patients was not the result of increased metabolism of the melatonin. It appeared that by some mechanism, the presence of cancer in the body reduced the ability of the pineal gland to produce melatonin.

One of their major contributions that has still not been fully explored is a study of the effect of other hormones produced by the pineal gland on cultured cancer cells in comparison to melatonin. They found the other hormones more effective in destroying a much larger range of cancers than melatonin. It seems strange to me that more effort to investigate these naturally occurring materials has not occurred to my knowledge. It is one of the reasons to believe that maximizing pineal output is preferable to trying to use melatonin pills.

One of their studies found a correlation between extent of suppression of melatonin and tumor size. It supports the notion that having cancer reduces melatonin production.

A number of their studies were concerned not with preventing cancer but in treating it with melatonin or with pineal extracts. Again they found that the extracts were more effective than melatonin. These studies included both animals and humans. They also looked into using melatonin along with other substances in treating cancer. Melatonin reduced side effects of chemotherapy.

Their most recent paper (2006) concerns the high incidence of breast and other cancers in the industrialized countries and how controlling environmental factors might help to bring down the rate. They discuss how maximizing the pineal production should be beneficial.

Summary:

1. Duration of light exposure and when melatonin is injected have a big effect on tumor growth in animals.

2. Reduced melatonin production in cancer patients (not enhanced removal) is the result of tumor growth.

3. Pineal hormones other than melatonin are more effective in destroying a much larger range of cancers than melatonin.

20

4. Melatonin concentration in blood and melatonin metabolite in urine are lower in patients with prostate cancer compared to those with benign prostate disease.

5. A reduction in cancer incidence may be possible by controlling the environmental factors known to reduce melatonin production.

CHAPTER 5
Richard G. Stevens, PhD

Dr. Stevens has been working for a long time trying to help figure out why people get cancer. One of his major interests has been in the possible role of iron overload. Largely on the basis of his work, published in the *Journal of the National Cancer Institute* and the *New England Journal of Medicine*, the Swedish food industry decided to cease iron fortification of flour in the early 1990s. A perplexing challenge, which Stevens began to engage in the late 1970s, is the confounding mystery of why breast cancer risk rises so dramatically as societies industrialize. He proposed in 1987 a radical new theory that use of electric lighting, resulting in lighted nights, might produce "circadian disruption," causing changes in the hormones relevant to breast cancer risk. Accumulating evidence has generally supported the idea, and it has received wide scientific and public attention. For example, his work has been featured on the covers of the popular weekly *Science News* (October 17, 1998) and the scientific journal *Cancer.*

The same year (2001) that Dr. Schernhammer published her breast cancer results for nurses working rotating shifts, Dr. Stevens published a study of a totally different group of women. This study aimed to discover whether working night shift increased the risk of breast cancer. They found an odds ratio of 1.6 (60% higher risk) for those working night shift compared to those who did not. It increased with the duration of night-shift work. A similar study of Norwegian women found an even higher odds ratio of 2.2 (120%) for women who worked night shift for 30 years.

For much of his earlier career, he had made studies of the effect of exposure to low-frequency magnetic fields. Some animal studies had seemed to show that these magnetic fields reduced melatonin flow just as light did. For the case of light, a mechanism tying melatonin to light existed. No such mechanism was offered for magnetic fields. Studies with humans had been far from convincing.

Dr. Stevens studied cancer rates in less-developed countries. He found that the breast cancer rate varies about fivefold between different societies. People from low-risk nations fairly quickly succumb to the very high rate when coming to an advanced country. Known risk factors only account for about a third of the cases of breast cancer. Light during the night may be the missing component.

Dr. Stevens's background in genetics served him well when he participated in a study with scientists at Yale University concerning variations in the Per3 gene. In this study, a length variant in the Per3 gene was found to be associated with a 1.7 odds ratio for breast cancer compared to women who did not have this variant. The Per3 gene is one of the genes associated with the circadian clock. This study included 389 women with breast cancer and 432 controls. The relationship between variations in the genes that make up the internal clock and cancer risk is pointing toward deeper understanding.

Dr. Stevens participated in a Finnish study in which the consistent duration of sleep was compared with incidence of breast cancer. This study showed that for consistently long sleepers (greater than 9 hours), the breast cancer rate was about one-fourth that of short sleepers (less than 6 hours). This is consistent with the thought that more time in darkness protects against breast cancer. Schernhammer had failed to find this to be the case for women in the Nurses' Health Study.

Another study done in Finland found a consistent decrease in the risk of breast cancer with increasing extent of visual impairment. This is in agreement with the hypothesis that exposure to light at night increases the risk of breast (and prostate) cancer. There were 17,557 individuals in the study.

A study of Long Island women compared shift work, exposure to light at home, and breast cancer incidence. This relatively small study (573 breast cancer patients) showed mixed results for the effect of working overnight shifts and of being exposed to light during the night at home. This points up the problem of finding individuals who are not exposed to light at night to act as controls. Everyone in our society is being exposed to light at night to some extent.

Summary of Dr. Stevens's main contributions:

1. Studies of night-shift workers found a significant increase in the risk of breast and prostate cancer compared to those not working at night.

2. His studies found a large difference in cancer rates between primitive and advanced societies.

3. Variants in certain genes associated with the circadian clock were found to correlate with the incidence of breast cancer.

4. Dr. Stephens was one of the scientists who participated in the committee that had the World Health Organization list shift work (which results in disruption of the circadian rhythm) as a probable carcinogen.

CHAPTER 6
William Hrushesky, MD and Patricia Wood, MD, PhD

Dr. Hrushesky and Dr. Wood are another husband-and-wife team of researchers who have jointly published more than 40 papers, with many other papers appearing under each of their names independently.

Dr. Hrushesky is a professor in the University of South Carolina School of Medicine Department of Developmental Biology and Anatomy and the Norman J. Arnold School of Public Health Department of Epidemiology and Biostatistics at Columbia, South Carolina. Dr. Hrushesky received a bachelor's degree with high honors in philosophy from Syracuse University Honors College in 1969, and an MD from the University of Buffalo Medical School in 1973.

Dr. Wood is also on the staff of South Carolina School of Medicine and also serves with the Veterans Administration. She received her several degrees at the University of Minnesota.

In the summary of an invited paper given in 2003 at the National Cancer Institute Office for Cancer Alternative and Complementary Medicine, Dr. Hrushesky said (in part),

> Circadian rhythms traverse all realms of biological organization. Circadian organization of the host-cancer balance is important to cancer prevention, screening,

diagnosis, and treatment. Melatonin, a hormone produced by the pineal gland, is a primary tuner, synchronizer, and chronobiotic that helps gate normal and cancer cells on a circadian basis.

Chronobiotics, synchronization, and tuning are different words for the ability to sharpen melatonin's amplitude and phase relationships through appropriately timed circadian interventions. This ability makes melatonin useful as a therapy for cancer prevention and treatment. Chronobiology and chronotherapy use timing to take advantage of robust endogenous synchronization.

Cellular proliferation and apoptosis, effects of hormones like melatonin, immune functions, and all other biological events are organized within circadian time. Circadian timing of short-half-life biological response modifiers such as the interferons, anticancer cytokines, and tumor necrosis factor can diminish or enhance tumor growth.

A group of circadian-clock control-genes that time events in the central circadian clock (suprachiasmatic nucleus) and also control every cell in the body were recently discovered and cloned. In mouse studies, mutations in one of these genes, mouse period 2, resulted in the spontaneous development of cancer."

Dr. Hrushesky's earliest studies were of kidney cancer. He found that drugs given to kill the cancer were less damaging to the kidney if given at certain times during the circadian cycle. This began a long career in which he and Dr. Wood sought to take advantage of the body's rhythm to optimize all kinds of interventions. They studied when, during a menstrual cycle, surgery for breast cancer resulted in the best outcome. They looked at other cycles such as summer or winter and even considered the effects of sun spot cycles.

They became best known for their work in optimizing the effects of chemotherapy by doing it at the optimum time during the circadian cycle. Optimum included not only the maximum damage to the cancer but also the least damage to the body and the least side effects. Much of this work was done using mice in which extremely detailed knowledge existed about how the genes controlled the production of various materials that in turn affected changes in other processes like cell division, DNA replication, cell propagation and how chemotherapy influenced this on a minute-by-minute basis.

One of their main concerns was that surgery had the effect of changing small tumors that were dormant into actively growing tumors. They became early proponents for caution in mammogram screening. They developed models to explain why the early screening (age 40) had little effect on mortality. These theories offer support to the concept of maximizing melatonin to destroy cancers in their microscopic stage before they grow. They also developed the powerful concept that there is a balance between cancer and the host that can be tipped one way or the other by lifestyle choices.

They have been pioneers in developing a more profound understanding of the mechanisms by which the genes control the details of the circadian cycle on a cellular and subcellular level and how this relates to both normal growth and the growth of cancer.

Summary of the work of Dr. Hrushesky and Dr. Wood

1. They demonstrated that circadian, seasonal, reproductive, and other cycles are preserved in individual cells within tissues and organs, including cancer cells.

2. They found that, essentially, interventions such as chemotherapy, radiation therapy, surgery, eating, and sleeping will all have

a range of effects depending on when in the circadian and other rhythms they occur.

3. They showed how the genes within each cell that make up its circadian clock control many aspects of normal and cancer cell activities and how this relates to the effectiveness of interventions.

4. They demonstrated that the time when melatonin is produced, controlled by the central clock in the suprachiasmatic nuclei (SCN), synchronizes daily cell-level circadian rhythms and that other means such as time of eating, may also serve that purpose.

5. They provided evidence that stabilizing the circadian cycle is a key to better health.

CHAPTER 7
Leonid Kayumov, PhD

Leonid Kayumov, PhD, DABSM, FAASM, Diplomate of the American Board of Sleep Medicine, received his PhD from Moscow University in the field of neuropsychology.

Currently he is director of the Sleep Research Laboratory at Toronto Western Hospital's University Health Network and an assistant professor of psychiatry at the University of Toronto. He is certified as a sleep disorders specialist by the American Board of Sleep Medicine. He has published extensively on all aspects of sleep medicine. He was involved in the preparation of several space expeditions designing special regimens for psychophysiological and physical training of cosmonauts, including express adaptation to the hypoxic conditions and sleep-wake patterns in different extreme situations. Main areas of his research interests include basic and clinical neurophysiology of the sleep-wake cycle, neuropharmacology and neuroendocrinology of circadian rhythm disorders, and impaired alertness and performance associated with shift work. He is doing pioneering research establishing a new field: holistic sleep medicine. He has established the Multimodal Alternative Treatment and Education Program (MATE) in Toronto Western Hospital, where he and his staff successfully use acupuncture, neuro-feedback, meditation, and art and music therapy for treatment of insomnia, anxiety, and depression. He has authored more than 100 research publications in the area of sleep medicine. On an academic front, he has participated in a number of research congresses and symposia including those in Moscow, Jerusalem, Warsaw, Berlin, Madrid, Washington DC, San Francisco, Istanbul, and Chicago. He is a member of the Israeli Association of Neuroscience and the American Academy of Sciences, and a fellow of the American Academy of Sleep Medicine.

Dr. Kayumov might not recognize himself as a "hero of breast cancer prevention research," but it was his 2005 study of the use of glasses that block blue light that established the principle that one does not have to go into darkness to initiate the flow of melatonin. This makes it not only possible but convenient to recover the full duration of melatonin flow (11–12 hours) that humans enjoyed during the time we evolved and which persisted up to the arrival of electric lighting. It is the longer flow of melatonin coupled with the ability to maintain a consistent circadian cycle that minimizes the risk of breast cancer. It wasn't until his 2007 paper that he voiced his belief that this method of blocking blue light reduced the risk of cancer. The paper is titled "Prevention of Melatonin Suppression by Nocturnal Lighting: Relevance to Cancer." He had subjects tested for melatonin during the night when kept in darkness. He then had them work a night shift under bright lights and found they produced very little melatonin. He next had them work a night shift under bright lights but with their eyes protected by blue-blocking glasses. Using glasses that blocked all light at wavelength shorter than 530nm resulted in only an 8% drop in melatonin compared to their night in darkness. These same conditions resulted in a 75% suppression of melatonin without the glasses. He described the use of glasses as a "cost effective, practical solution to the problem of increased malignancy rates in shift workers."

Here we have another example in which even the author of the paper does not apparently recognize that this doesn't just affect the cancer rate in shift workers. It affects the cancer risk in anyone who is exposed to light in the evening. It applies to everyone who is robbed of the 11 to 12 hours of melatonin flow known to be possible, by exposure to evening light.

In subsequent papers, he turned his attention away from cancer to the effect of melatonin on mood disorders and depression and to the use of light therapy, along with exercise, in weight and body-fat reduction.

Summary of Dr. Kayumov's work:

His major contribution to breast cancer prevention was his discovery that blocking the blue light known to suppress melatonin restored its flow during the night.

CHAPTER 8
Vladimir Anisimov, MD, PhD, DSc

Dr. Anisimov is one of the pioneers of the study of the pineal gland. He began his studies of the effect of extracts from the pineal gland on various cancers in the 1970s. He spent his entire career at the Petrov Research Institute for Oncology in St. Petersburg, Russia. Control of the Institute passed from one government agency to another and physically had to be rebuilt after being destroyed and then moved at least once to a new location. During those tumultuous years in Russian history, he managed to continue producing over one hundred papers concerning cancer. Sixty-three papers appear in a PubMed search of his name and melatonin. His experimental work was largely done using rats and mice, but he also did studies of cultures of human breast cancer cell lines.

A number of his earlier papers concerned the beneficial effect of melatonin on aging. He found that melatonin greatly extended the life of fruit flies and slowed the aging process in some mammals. Much of the earlier excitement concerning these studies faded as it failed to translate into a "fountain of youth."

He did many studies showing the benefit of melatonin in preventing or slowing down tumor growth in rats and mice. He demonstrated the benefit of long periods of darkness in maximizing melatonin and the harmful effects of prolonged light exposure.

He was also one of the earliest to demonstrate the relationship between the genes controlling the circadian clock and cancer.

While many of his studies focused on breast cancer, a recent paper looked at the effect of light duration on chemically induced colon cancer in rats. He found that the number of tumors and the stage and invasiveness of the tumors all increased with light duration and decreased with light deprivation.

In another fairly recent paper he reported the effect on general health and spontaneous cancer development in male rats of different light schedules, including 12 hours light– 12 hours darkness, continuous light, and natural light in northwest Russia. He found that both natural light and continuous light accelerated aging and the development of tumors compared to the 12:12 schedule. He found that including melatonin in drinking water impeded the start and growth of tumors in the continuous and natural light conditions.

In a second paper, he did the same experiment with female rats with similar results. For the male rats the spontaneous cancers were primarily liver cancers, while in the female rats they were primarily mammary cancers. Again the 12:12 light cycle was protective, as was melatonin added to drinking water in the natural and continuous light conditions.

All of his studies in rats and mice appeared to confirm the findings of others concerning humans: that maximizing melatonin by controlling light reduced risk of cancer, while excessive exposure to light was detrimental in terms of accelerated aging and cancer development.

Summary of the wok of Dr. Anisimov:

1. In a large number of animal studies with rats and mice, He found that long exposure to light increased the incidence of cancer (both spontaneous and induced) while controlling light to maximize melatonin decreased incidence and slowed growth. Long periods of light increased aging and the incidence of cancer.

2. Maximizing natural melatonin was beneficial in reducing cancer risk. Introducing melatonin externally was beneficial if naturally produced melatonin was absent due to light exposure.

CHAPTER 9
The Research Staff at the University of Cantabria

In the 1990s, a group at the Medical School at the University of Cantabria, Spain, published many studies of the effect of melatonin on cultured breast cancer cells. The cell line they were studying is responsive to estrogen. They found that the inhibition of cell growth by melatonin was dependent on the presence of estrogen. They discovered in one study that the inhibition of cell growth by melatonin was most marked if the concentration varied in a manner as it would in a person; that is in a 24-hour rhythm where it increased and decreased during one 12-hour period and was absent in the next twelve-hour period.

In another experiment, they found that the inhibition of growth of cultured human breast cancer cells only occurred for fast-growing cells. In another study, they concluded that one mechanism by which melatonin inhibited growth of human breast cancer cells in culture was by blocking DNA synthesis. In another study, they identified the details by which melatonin reduced the invasive character of human breast cancer cells. This was a result of decreasing both the attachment and motility of the cells by changes in certain genes.

Breast cancer cells have an ability to use an enzyme action to produce estrogen, which then stimulates their growth. This is called aromatase action. A further benefit of melatonin was discovered in its ability to inhibit the aromatase (enzyme) action of human breast cancer cells in producing estrogen, which in turn stimulates growth. Other aromatase inhibitors are used in breast cancer prevention. This is in addition to melatonin's ability to reduce estrogen production in the ovaries and its ability to block estrogen receptors. This makes melatonin a complete anti-estrogen drug.

Although the majority of the papers from the group[at the University of Cantabria concerned experiments with human breast cancers in culture, they did a study in which they looked at the effect of dim light during darkness on chemically induced mammary tumors in rats. Tumor growth was increased, estradiol levels in serum were high, and excretion of melatonin metabolite in urine was reduced. The interesting sidelight was their use of very dim light in apparent recognition of the extremely high sensitivity of rats' eyes to light. It evidently includes the sensors that control the circadian cycle as well as the rods and cones that produce vision.

To test the aromatase-inhibiting ability of melatonin in animals, the group studied rats whose ovaries had been removed to exclude estrogen normally produced by the ovaries. Mammary tumors were induced chemically, and testosterone was injected. Without melatonin, the tumors generated estrogen from testosterone by aromatase action that stimulated tumor growth. Animals also provided with melatonin had reduced tumor growth and reduced estrogen as anticipated. What had occurred in culture also occurred in live animals. In another study, they found that melatonin enhances the aromatase action of the well-known aromatase inhibitor aminoglutethimide used in treating metastatic breast cancer.

Cadmium is well known as a carcinogen. Its action depends partially on its ability to mimic estrogen. In studies with mice, they found that melatonin can blunt the damage of cadmium just as it does with estrogen. Protecting the body from heavy metals like cadmium is another reason to maximize natural melatonin.

In a different but related experiment, the group looked at the effect of melatonin and estrogen supplementation in female rats that had their ovaries removed to emulate postmenopausal women. The controls showed large weight gain not observed in the treated animals. By including melatonin, the increased risk of breast cancer is avoided while obtaining the benefits of hormone supplementation. They suggest that clinical trials in postmeno- pausal women would be appropriate, especially in view of the epidemic nature of obesity.

Their accomplishments in demonstrating the benefits of melato- nin are summed up in their own words as follows:

> Melatonin exerts oncostatic (cancer-killing) effects on different kinds of tumors, especially on hormone- dependent (estrogen) breast cancer....Melatonin inhibits the growth of breast cancer...through three different mechanisms: (a) the indirect neuroendocrine mechanism, which includes the melatonin down-regulation of the hypothalamic-pituitary-reproductive axis and the consequent reduction of circulating levels of gonadal (ovarian) estrogens, (b) direct melatonin actions at tumor cell level by interacting with (blocking)) the activation of the estrogen receptor, thus behaving as a selective estrogen receptor modulator (SERM), and (c) the regulation of the enzymes involved in the biosynthesis of estrogens in peripheral tissues, thus behaving as a selective estrogen enzyme modulator (SEEM)....Thus, a single molecule has both SERM and SEEM properties, one of the main objectives desired for the breast antitumoral drugs. Since the inhibition of enzymes involved in the biosynthesis of estrogens is currently one of the first therapeutic strategies used against the growth of breast cancer, melatonin modulation of different enzymes involved in the synthesis of steroid hormones (estrogens) makes, collectively, this indolamine (melatonin) an interesting anticancer drug in the prevention and treatment of estrogen-dependent mammary tumors.

Summary of the main contributions of the group at the University of Cantabria:

1. They provided a detailed picture of how melatonin controls the cancer-promoting effect of estrogen in three distinct ways and its

benefit in inhibiting estrogen responsive cancers. Seventy percent of cancers are responsive to estrogen.

2. They demonstrated the possible benefits of a combination of hormone replacement therapy and melatonin for avoiding obesity in post-menopausal women.

3. They demonstrated the damaging effects of light at night in promoting breast cancer growth in rats.

CHAPTER 10
Russel J. Reiter, MD, PhD

Dr. Reiter might be correctly referred to as Dr. Melatonin. He has spent a lifetime studying this molecule and its wondrous effects on living things. A University of Texas publication describes him in the follow words:

> Dr. Reiter teaches in the Medical Neuroscience and Dental Microscopic Anatomy courses at the Health Science Center. He also gives lectures in the History of Anatomy, Introduction to Research and in Journal Clubs of several departments. He is the Editor-in-Chief of the Journal of Pineal Research and on the Editorial Board of 7 other journals. He is the recipient of numerous awards including three honorary doctor of medicine degrees and, most recently, the Presidential Distinguished Scholar Award from UTHSCSA.
>
> Dr. Reiter's research interests relate to free radical aspects of disease processes and aging. Of particular interest is defining the role of oxygen derivatives in neurodegenerative diseases and their function in apoptosis, necrosis and neuronal degeneration. These studies typically involve measurements of oxidatively damaged polyunsaturated fatty acids, proteins and DNA.
>
> Besides investigating the functional relevance of free radicals to age-associated organ deterioration, Dr. Reiter's group is investigating the free radical scavenging

and antioxidant properties of pineal indoleamines, most notably melatonin. The investigations include the mechanisms of interaction of melatonin with free radicals and the resulting products. These studies have utilized thermodynamic analyses, electron ionization mass spectroscopy, nuclear magnetic resonance, high-performance liquid chromotography, electron spin resonance spectroscopy and biochemical and molecular biological techniques to unravel the processes involved. This research group is also investigating the role of melatonin as an antitoxin against a variety of xenobiotics and environmental pollutants and the functional significance of melatonin and other indoleamines with processes of aging.

Dr. Reiter has written 1064 scientific articles that are abstracted on PubMed.gov, the US government's medical database. If one adds the word melatonin to his name in the search box, the number of papers listed drops to 802. This is a measure of his focus on this substance. If one adds pineal to his name the result it 544 papers. His first papers referenced in PubMed (1964) concern kidney damage in rats. In 1965 his first paper concerning melatonin and the pineal gland is entitled "Pineal Gland: Influence on Gonads of Male Hamsters."

One of Dr. Reiter's major contributions to cancer prevention research is that he trained some of those mentioned in this book when they were his students. If we search PubMed with the names Reiter RJ and Blask DE, we find 30 papers, the first of which is from 1973. This relationship evidently continued over about 10 years. If one searches the names of Reiter and Brainard together, one finds 16 papers, the first of which was from 1980 and continued over about six years. Blask and Brainard did not publish together at that time but did publish seven papers together starting in 1999 and continuing for ten years. It was during the time that Blask and Brainard were students of Reiter that the powerful effect of the duration of light and darkness on the reproductive and other hormones was first observed and the role that the pineal gland played in all of it. The experimental techniques for working with small mammals that were developed in those years equipped these men to solve many of the puzzles concerning how light and darkness affect health.

In 1995 Dr. Reiter along with writer Jo Robinson produced the book *Melatonin* that was distributed by Bantam Books. The cover contained the following:

Breakthrough Discoveries
That Can Help You
Combat Aging
Boost Your Immune System
Reduce Your Risk of Cancer
and Heart Disease
Get a Better Night's Sleep

While there is a great deal of evidence that the above statements are all true, the book tended to present the information in a slightly sensational manner. Another book appeared about the same time by Walter Pierpaoli, MD, PhD, and others that was even more enthusiastic. It is entitled *The Melatonin Miracle: Nature's Age-Reversing, Disease-Fighting, Sex-Enhancing Hormone*. This was picked up by the media and hyped with the promise of no more aging. Melatonin was described as the "fountain of youth." It ended up with melatonin being discredited in the minds of many people. This points out a danger of going public with scientific discoveries. Dr. Reiter authored 10 other more scholarly books that further document his immense contribution to our knowledge about the pineal gland and melatonin.

In 1997 a conference was convened in Germany to discuss the pineal gland and cancer. The proceedings of this conference were published with the title "The Pineal Gland and Cancer" by Springer-Verlag in 2000. . It was edited by Dr. Bartsch and included Dr. Reiter as one of the contributing authors. Dr. Reiter described how melatonin can help to prevent cancer by protecting cells from damage to their DNA by oxidative species or free radicals. Unlike other antioxidants, melatonin can enter the nucleus of the cell where DNA damage can occur. By neutralizing the free radicals, damage to the DNA is avoided, thus reducing the risk of cancer. This is at the center of the argument in favor of maximizing the time that melatonin should be present in the bloodstream to reduce the risk of cancer.

While the above refers to how melatonin prevents the start of a cancer, it reduces the risk of cancer through a host of different mechanisms that are summarized in a recent paper (2010) by Dr. Reiter and others. They are enumerated in the quote from the abstract of that paper as follows:

> The objective of the present article is to offer a global
> and integrative view of the mechanisms involved in
> the oncostatic actions of this indoleamine. Due to the
> wide spectrum of melatonin's actions, the mechanisms
> that may be involved in its ability to counteract tumor
> growth are varied. These include: a) antioxidant effects;
> b) regulation of the estrogen receptor expression and
> transactivation; c) modulation of the enzymes involved
> in the local synthesis of estrogens; d) modulation of
> cell cycle and induction of apoptosis; e) inhibition
> of telomerase activity; f) inhibition of metastasis; g)
> prevention of circadian disruption; h) antiangiogenesis;
> i) epigenetic effects; j) stimulation of cell differentiation;
> and k) activation of the immune system. The data
> supporting each of these oncostatic actions of melatonin
> are summarized in this review. Moreover, the list of
> actions described may not be exhaustive in terms of how
> melatonin modulates tumor growth.

Much of the meaning of the above paragraph is obscured by the use of highly technical terms. I will attempt to translate the above into terms the average reader will understand: (a) antioxi-dant effects are the ability to eliminate free radicals; (b) melatonin has the ability to block the cancer stimulating effect of estrogen; (c) some tumors have the ability to stimulate the production of estrogen right near the tumor, and melatonin blocks this process; (d) melatonin interferes with cancer cell function, leading to cell death; (e) telomerase activity allows cancer cells to become immortal, and melatonin blocks this process; (f) melatonin blocks the spread of cancer cells to distant places where they form new tumors; (g) avoiding interruption of the normal daily schedule helps prevent cancer; (h) melatonin helps block the formation of new blood vessels needed to supply the growing tumor; (i) melatonin blocks the cancer-promoting action of certain genes; (j) the process by which immature cells become mature cells is accelerated in the presence of melatonin and (k) melatonin helps activate the immune system.

The above is from Dr. Reiter's most recent paper concerning cancer and how melatonin reduces its risk. The following is from the abstract from the first paper that appears on a PubMed search of his name plus cancer, titled "Breast Cancer, Blindness and Melatonin."

Eur J Cancer. 1992;28(2-3):501-3.

Breast cancer, blindness and melatonin.

Coleman MP, Reiter RJ.

Source

Unit of Descriptive Epidemiology, International Agency for Research on Cancer, Lyon, France.

Abstract

The hypothesis is advanced that blindness from an early age may lead to a reduced risk of breast cancer through altered patterns of melatonin secretion by the pineal gland. The available experimental evidence in animals and in vitro is consistent with this hypothesis. The hypothesis can be tested in humans by a simple observational study in which the breast cancer risk in blind women is compared with that of all women. The effect of age at onset, duration and degree of blindness could also be assessed, after adjustment for known risk factors for breast cancer. Melatonin might prove to be a natural oncostatic agent of practical value in cancer prevention.

At about the same time that Dr. Reiter was suggesting the experiment with blind women, Hahn (see below) was carrying it out with the results shown in this abstract for the article titled "Profound Bilateral Blindess and the Incidence of Breast Cancer."

Epidemiology. 1991 May;2(3):208-10.

Profound bilateral blindness and the incidence of breast cancer.

Hahn RA.

Source

Division of Surveillance and Epidemiologic Studies, Centers for Disease Control, Atlanta, GA 30333.

Abstract

This case-control study addressed the hypothesis that uninterrupted exposure to light is associated with increased rates of breast cancer. We compared the odds of profound binocular blindness among women with a diagnosis of breast cancer with the odds of profound binocular blindness among women with diagnoses of coronary heart disease or stroke. All hospital discharges in the National Hospital Discharge Survey from 1979 through 1987 were analyzed, after exclusion of women with diabetes. Profoundly blind women were half as likely to have breast cancer as women who were not profoundly blind. This effect diminished substantially with increasing age.

These results for blind women were confirmed in later studies both in Europe and the United States. They suggest that if a woman would avoid blue light for a number of hours before bedtime, she could maximize her melatonin and reduce her risk to that of blind women—in other words, cut her risk in half.

Dr. Reiter's earliest work relating directly to cancer looked at the possible increase in cancer associated with the exposure to varying magnet fields such as produced by power lines. Because of the relatively high conductivity of water, the electric fields that are also produced by ordinary power lines do not penetrate the body to any depth. However, the magnetic fields do penetrate. How they interact with the body is not completely clear. Magnetic fields might interact with the electric currents that flow in nerve fibers. The EKG we are all familiar with measures these currents produced in connection with the beating of the heart. Some studies with small animals had shown a drop in nighttime melatonin as a result of exposure to these fields. Dr. Reiter proposed that this might be a mechanism for an increased cancer rate. The most recent studies (April 2012, not by Dr. Reiter) showed no decrease in melatonin in rats due to exposure to a 60-hertz magnetic field of one gauss for 30 days. The fact that some studies seemed to show a drop in melatonin due to a magnetic field might be explained by the drop in melatonin due to exposure to light. Because rats' eyes are so extremely sensitive to light, just light coming through a crack under a closed laboratory door might have been the actual cause for the reduction of melatonin.

I have my own theory for the alleged increase in the cancer rate associated with living next to power lines. Power lines are kept free of the growth of vegetation by aerial spraying with herbicides. Some herbicides are known to be carcinogens.

One of the main themes in Dr. Reiter's work is the protection from cancer due to the antioxidant properties of melatonin. In a 2000 paper entitled "Increased Levels of Oxidatively Damaged DNA Induced by Chromium (III) and H2O2: Protection by Melatonin and Related Molecules," he showed how this can be applied. He further demonstrated how the antioxidant properties of melatonin provided protection of the body from damage caused by exposure to ionizing radiation such as X-rays and cosmic rays.

In a 2001 paper entitled "Comparison of the Protective Effect of Melatonin with Other Antioxidants in the Hamster Kidney Model of Estradiol-Induced DNA Damage," Dr. Reiter showed how melatonin protects the kidney from cancer-initiating DNA damage.

Another interesting study looked at whether the exposure to ionizing radiation used in radiotherapy for brain cancer would reduce the ability of the pineal gland (located in the head) to produce melatonin. While he observed a large variation in the amount of melatonin produced by different people, he found no evidence that radiotherapy reduced the production of melatonin.

This abstract of Dr. Reiter's 2002 paper "Potential Biological Consequences of Excessive Light Exposure: Melatonin Suppression, DNA Damage, Cancer and Neurodegenerative Diseases" is printed in full. It is a clear, easy-to-understand indictment of the use of light at night. It makes one wonder how much longer it will take before the medical community begins warning people of this ubiquitous danger.

This brief review summarizes some of the biological effects of light exposure at an inappropriate time (during the normal dark period) and the potential negative physiological consequences of this light exposure. Two major systems are significantly influenced by light at night. Thus, the circadian system and melatonin synthesis are altered when light is extended into the normal dark period or when the dark period is interrupted by light. This summary reviews the potential sequelae of chronic inappropriate light exposure and the suppression of endogenous melatonin levels. Given that melatonin is a free radical scavenger and antioxidant, conditions that involve free radical damage may be aggravated by light suppression of melatonin levels. The conditions of particular interest for this review are excessive DNA damage (which potentially leads to cancer), cellular destruction in neurodegenerative diseases and aging itself. Further research should be conducted to more accurately define the potential negative impact of light at abnormal times on animal and human pathophysiology.

A 2004 paper reviews the ways in which melatonin may protect the body from ionizing radiation that occurs during X-ray imaging, computer-aided tomography, and emission from radioactive species (e.g., nuclear accidents). Because it is free from significant side effects even in large doses, it is puzzling (to the author at least) why it is not a common practice to use it in connection with these procedures.

In 2005 Dr. Reiter reported the results of a study of the effectiveness of melatonin in treating two different cell lines of prostate cancer. Both were inhibited in growth, and cell differentiation was enhanced. Because the production of melatonin tends to decrease with age and prostate cancer occurs in old age, melatonin supplementation would seem to be in order. In any event, it makes sense to maximize the time when melatonin is present in the body by avoiding blue light in the hours before bedtime.

In a very recent paper (June 2012) entitled "Melatonin Uses in Oncology: Breast Cancer Prevention and Reduction of the Side Effects of Chemotherapy and Radiation," Dr. Reiter reviews all the ways melatonin can be beneficial in preventing and treating cancer. He states, in part, "The clinical utility of melatonin depends on the appropriate identification of its actions. Because of its SERM (selective estrogen receptor modulators) and SEEM (selective estrogen enzyme modulators) properties, and its virtual absence of contraindications, melatonin could be an excellent adjuvant with the drugs currently used for breast cancer prevention (antiestrogens and antiaromatases). The antioxidant actions also make melatonin a suitable treatment to reduce oxidative stress associated with chemotherapy, especially with anthracyclines, and radiotherapy."

Summary of Dr. Reiter's contribution to cancer prevention:

1. He and his students developed many techniques for working with small animals that allowed the discovery of the benefits of melatonin in cancer prevention.

2. He engendered an interest in how melatonin benefits health in his students who became some of the heroes described in this book.

3. He identified many of the complex ways in which melatonin helps to fight against the development of cancer.

4. Through his book *Melatonin,* he helped educate ordinary people about the many benefits to health of melatonin.

CHAPTER 11
Others

There are many other heroes of cancer prevention research who we really need to honor for their contributions but for whom a whole chapter does not seem appropriate. We will name a few who contributed in some significant way.

As early as 1978, a paper by M. Cohen, M. Lippman, and B. Chabner entitled "Role of the Pineal Gland in Aetiology and Treatment of Breast Cancer" spelled out very clearly some of the main evidence that the pineal gland and melatonin play a significant role in breast cancer. Because of the clarity, I'm including the abstract without changes. Note that this was more than 34 years ago.

> The hypothesis that diminished function of the pineal gland may promote the development of breast cancer in human beings is suggested by the relation between breast cancer and prolonged oestrogen [English spelling] excess, and by the observation that the pineal secretion, melatonin, inhibits ovarian oestrogen production, pituitary gonadotrophin production, and sexual development and maturation. The hypothesis is supported by the following points. (1) Pineal calcification is commonest in countries with high rates of breast cancer and lowest in areas with a low incidence; the incidences of pineal calcification and of breast cancer are moderate among the black population in the United States. (2) Chlorpromazine raises serum-melatonin; there are reports that psychiatric patients taking chlorpromazine have a lower incidence of breast cancer. (3) Although information is lacking on

breast cancer, the pineal and melatonin may influence tumour induction and growth in experimental animals. (4) The demonstration of a melatonin receptor in human ovary suggests a direct influence of this hormone on the ovarian function, and possibly oestrogen production. (5) Impaired pineal secretion is believed to be an important factor triggering puberty (early menarche is a risk factor for breast cancer).

In a 1982 paper by L. S. Kothari, P. N. Shah, and M. C. Mhatre with the title "Effect of Continuous Light on the Incidence of 9,10-Dimethyl-1,2-Benzanthracene Induced Mammary Tumors in Female Holtzman Rats," they observed that 95% of the rats developed tumors compared to only 60% for rats raised under 10 hours of light and 14 hours of darkness. The time to develop tumors was also reduced by the continuous light. The continuous light prevented the production of melatonin.

In a 1983 paper by L. R. Stanberry, T. K. Das Gupta, and C. W. Beattie titled "Photoperiodic Control of Melanoma Growth in Hamsters: Influence of Pinealectomy and Melatonin," they describe how changing from 10 to 18 hours of darkness decreased tumor growth rate. Pinealectomy increased the tumor growth rate. This is one of the earliest reported cases showing the benefit of long hours of darkness. Unfortunately this work was not continued by these authors.

In a 1994 paper by R. J. Nelson and J. M. Blom titled "Photoperiodic Effects on Tumor Development and Immune Function," they write (in part) in the abstract as follows:

> Adult female deer mice (Peromyscus maniculatus) were housed in either long (LD 16:8) or short (LD 8:16) days for 8 weeks, then injected with the chemical carcinogen 9,10-dimethyl-1,2-benzanthracene (DMBA) dissolved in dimethyl sulfoxide (DMSO) or with the DMSO vehicle alone. Animals were evaluated weekly for 8 weeks after injection. None of the animals treated with DMSO developed tumors in any of the experiments. Nearly 90%

of the long-day deer mice injected with DMBA developed squamous cell carcinoma. *None of the short-day deer mice injected with DMBA developed tumors.*

(The bold type and *italics* are mine.)

This is a remarkable result. The only thing changed was the length of the dark period during which melatonin could flow. If nothing else will convince you to wear blue-blocking glasses(or use special light bulbs), this alone should convince you.

A 2006 paper by a group of 16 epidemiologists at the University of Occupational and Environmental Health, Kitakyushu, Japan, found that compared with day workers, rotating-shift workers were at a significantly increased risk for prostate cancer (relative risk = 3.0), whereas fixed-night work was associated with a small and nonsignificant increase in risk. This report is the first known to reveal a significant relation between rotating-shift work and prostate cancer. This was in a study of more than 14,000 men.

In a paper published in 2006 by K. J. Navara and R. J. Nelson titled "The Dark Side of Light at Night: Physiological, Epidemiological, and Ecological Consequences," they write in the abstract as follows:

Organisms must adapt to the temporal characteristics of their surroundings to successfully survive and reproduce. Variation in the daily light cycle, for example, acts through endocrine and neurobiological mechanisms to control several downstream physiological and behavioral processes. Interruptions in normal circadian light cycles and the resulting disruption of normal melatonin rhythms cause widespread disruptive effects involving multiple body systems, the results of which can have serious medical consequences for individuals, as well as large-scale ecological implications for populations. With the invention of electric lights about a century ago, the temporal organization of the environment has been drastically altered for many species, including humans.

In addition to the incidental exposure to light at night through light pollution, humans also engage in increasing amounts of shift-work, resulting in repeated and often long-term circadian disruption. The increasing prevalence of exposure to light at night has significant social, ecological, behavioral, and health consequences that are only now becoming apparent. This review addresses the complicated web of potential behavioral and physiological consequences resulting from exposure to light at night, as well as the large-scale medical and ecological implications that may result.

A 2001 study by E. B. Klerman, J. M. Zeitzer, J. F. Duffy, S. B. Khalsa, and C. A. Czeisler (from Harvard Medical School) found that totally blind people produced melatonin for about 9 to 11 hours. People with normal vision who were kept in the dark had about the same duration of melatonin flow.

In 2008, H. J. Burgess and L. F. Fogg published the results of a study of melatonin flow during darkness for 85 men and 85 women by sampling saliva every 30 minutes. There were considerable differences in both the amount of melatonin produced and the duration. The average duration was about 11.5 hours. This is somewhat longer than the average found in the smaller study mentioned above. The big difference between the 6 or 7 hours of darkness the average American experiences and the 11 -12 hours known to be possible, is quite striking. We are only producing about half of the melatonin we could be getting by simply avoiding blue light in the evening.

A 2009 study by I. Kloog, A. Haim, R. G. Stevens, M. Barchana, and B. A. Portnov found that for women in Israel, the incidence of breast cancer showed a positive correlation with the luminance (brightness) of their community measured by a satellite in space. No such correlation existed for the incidence of lung cancer. In a subsequent study, they looked for a correlation between luminance of the community and lung cancer, colon cancer, and prostate cancer in men in communities throughout the world. They found a positive correlation with prostate cancer but not for lung or colon cancer. These findings are consistent with the facts that both breast and prostate cancers are known to be stimulated by estrogen, melatonin suppresses the effects of estrogen, and light suppresses melatonin. These findings support the idea of blocking blue light at night to reduce the incidence of both breast and prostate cancer.

CHAPTER 12
Conclusions

After looking at the work of all these scientists, some readers might have come to believe that reducing the risk of breast and prostate cancer is an extremely complicated business and that no simple action is going to be possible. I believe quite the opposite. All of the studies point to the same conclusions. I'll try to state them as simply as I can.

Short Version.:

Using light at night reduces the time when melatonin can be present in your body. Melatonin fights cancer in many ways and helps promote good sleep that is vital for good health. It is primarily the blue component in ordinary white light that causes melatonin suppression. Using light bulbs that don't make blue light or wearing eyeglasses that block it for several hours before a regular bedtime will restore full protection. Getting up at the same time every day and exposing the eyes to ordinary white light will help lock in the circadian cycle. Exercise and exposing the eyes to lots of light during the day have both been shown in other studies to increase the amount of melatonin produced at night.

A Longer Version.:

1. The pineal gland and a stable circadian cycle are very important to health.

2. Cells throughout the body have circadian clocks that are synchronized by the central circadian clock located in the SCN.

3. The central circadian clock is kept in synchronization with the clock on the wall by exposure of the eyes to light in the morning.

4. Special cells in the retina (that are different from the rods and cones that produce vision) connect to the circadian clock. These special cells respond most strongly to blue light.

5. By blocking blue light with amber glasses, the body acts as if in darkness (virtual darkness).

6. At approximately the same time every day, the circadian clock will stimulate the pineal gland to start producing melatonin, but only if the eyes are in darkness.

7. The average duration of the flow of melatonin is about 11.5 hours per night if in darkness . Because of exposure to both natural and artificial light, the duration is much less for most Americans.

8. Exposing the eyes to light in the evening delays the start of the flow of melatonin.

9. Melatonin is a powerful cancer fighter. It blunts the cancer-promoting effect of estrogen in three ways: it reduces production by the ovaries, avoids stimulating tumor growth by blocking estrogen receptors, and prevents enzyme action at cells that produce estrogen (works as an aromatase inhibitor). Melatonin blocks the metabolism of linoleic acid by cancer cells. The result of metabolism of linoleic acid is a material that stimulates metastasis. Melatonin thus inhibits metastasis. Melatonin also keeps the body from producing blood vessels that provide nutrients to tumors. Melatonin is a powerful antioxidant that helps the body to destroy cells with damaged DNA.

Action Plan:

Both men and women should either switch to safe light bulbs (that block blue light) at night or start wearing glasses that block blue light for a few hours before a consistent bedtime. Without action, knowledge is of little value.